Unapologetic Leadership

Finding The Moral Courage To Do The Right Thing.

DR. KWADWO KYEREMANTENG

WITH LINDA HULME LEAHY

KWADWO KYEREMANTENG

1977
Kwadwo Kyeremanteng born Oct. 3, General Hospital, Edmonton.

1995
Graduates from Archbishop MacDonald Secondary School. Off to the University of Alberta.

2001
Meets Cathy Ogilvie as he tends bar. They marry in 2007.

2005
Moves to Ottawa to begin residency.

2012
Critical Care and Palliative Physician at Ottawa Hospital.

2012
Son number 1, Teddy.

2014
Son number 2, Marlow.

2017
Senior Clinician Investigator, Ottawa Hospital Research Institute.

2018
Dad, Solomon dies.

2018
Son number 3, Ezekiel.

2019
Creates Solving Healthcare podcast: Kwadcast.

2019
Early Career Researcher of The Year, University of Ottawa.

2021
Department Head, Critical Care, The Ottawa Hospital

2023
Solving Healthcare With Dr. K debuts Sauga 960 Radio.

2023
Unapologetic Leadership: Finding The Moral Courage To Do The Right Thing.

Dedication:

To my mom who showed me how to love and find happiness in every endeavour.

To my siblings, especially the boys who always made me smile, thank you for being my constant companions and for making my childhood so special.

To my children, I hope one day you will find in this book a roadmap to an unapologetic and authentic life.

To Catherine, my rock through all the craziness.

Finally, to my father, Solomon Kyeremanteng who gifted me with the principles for courageous and unapologetic living.

Kwadwo Kyeremanteng, August, 2023.

Credits:

Front and back cover photos: Jenny Payne Photography.

Cover and Interior Design: Ken Cadinouche.

Table of Contents

Note: Some of the content of this book came from the Kwadcast.
Those elements are italicized.

Foreword

Growing up, my husband, Kwadwo, was taught a principle by his father Solomon: always do more than anyone else to ensure you're not overlooked because of your skin colour.

I saw this principle in action for the first 20 years we were together. I did not always attribute it to his fight against inequality and the prejudice he faced through direct and systemic racism. Often it came across as an ethic of hard work, dedication, and competitiveness, all principles that I admired in him.

However, as the years progressed and we all gained more insights on the experiences of ourselves, our peers, and the influences of racism in the systems we work, play and live in, we began to understand the underpinnings of this drive. These underpinnings were based in fear. Fear of judgment, prejudice, and discrimination. Fear that his hard work would not take him as far as he wanted to go, as far as he deserved to go. Solomon's principle was a response to the painful reality of systemic racism. Instead of society championing fairness, the marginalized are often asked to turn the burden of prejudice into fuel for their drive.

Kwadwo is no stranger to fear. Every person of colour who has faced racial profiling or felt the weight of racial prejudice understands it. But he learned to navigate these challenges without voicing them. He encountered these inequities in many areas, from the hockey rink as a young child to higher education and healthcare systems. Whether it was being one of the few black faces in medical school photos, being passed up for a work-related opportunity, or facing subtle or overt racial biases in interactions with colleagues and patients, he learned to navigate carefully. He often remarked, "I have to be careful here. I know I'm playing short-handed, but it's not like I can 'play the race card'. I have to show these guys I have more game than everyone else."

But this fear-based approach takes its toll. It is stressful to always be vigilant and never truly your full self. Kwadwo had been feeling this toll for a while. He was tired of playing this game. So, just a few months prior to the pandemic, he started his podcast, Solving Healthcare. The podcast was something he could do on his own terms, "unapologetically", and gave him the experience of what it was like to be his true self AND a doctor. Then the onset of the COVID pandemic followed by the Black Lives Matter movement propelled everything forward.

When COVID hit, he had a very different experience in the ICU than what was being portrayed in the media. Don't get me wrong, we were all afraid at the start. Would this be like SARS? Would he get sick? Bring it home to the family? There were so many unknowns, but he told me "This is what I signed up for. It is why I chose to be a doctor, to be an intensivist. It's my duty." And over time, maybe earlier than others because of his direct exposure to the virus, we began to see more nuance in the story. Fear-based decision making is like having blinders on. You cannot see all the potential consequences of your decisions. Your view is narrowed in on what you are afraid of. Fear of infection was not the only message needed here. And if decisions were going to be made through fear, they were going to negatively impact people in a lot more ways than this virus could.

We watched as it became clear that marginalized communities were suffering disproportionately from these fear-based decisions. These communities, often frontline workers, had a contrasting experience to those who were able to shelter in place and keep their jobs during lockdowns (including those who were making the decisions). Kwadwo had a strong drive to say something to support these communities, and all people who were suffering the consequences of COVID-related restrictions. He supported a more balanced approach, which considered the whole spectrum of health implications of decisions made during this time: the immediate risk of infection as well as the short and long-term implications for people have reduced or, in some cases, no access to health, mental health, and social services, one that considered what we have always known to be the most important determinants of population health like income, education, socialization and community and physical activity.

This was an unpopular opinion throughout the pandemic, but Kwadwo chose not to merely fit in or stay silent. Instead, he led unapologetically, embracing his identity and mission amid the prevailing uncertainty. With the murder of George Floyd and the triggering of the Black Lives Matter movement, he found more strength and courage to speak up. It was time to start leading authentically.

Contrary to the fears that constrained him during most of his education and training, this time, his boldness did not hold him back. On the contrary, it propelled him forward. He started taking more action at work, moving forward more quickly with ideas for research and projects that actually "move the needle" in patient care. This move toward bolder action did not go unnoticed. He became Chief of ICU, founded Solving Healthcare Media, and saw a surge in his online influence.

He built a community of visionary leaders and frequently appeared on national broadcasts.

Kwadwo has always maintained an unwavering ethic of hard work and has always had a magnetic personality. But now it is different. When he chose to live with authenticity, act in alignment with his values, without apology, he flourished. Not just in terms of career success, but in his own measures of true success, doing the right thing and making a tangible difference in everything that he does, and most importantly he has flourished in himself. It is not that he is immune to fear. But now he responds to it, not by running from it or changing himself, but by embracing it and using it as a signal that whatever he is doing may be hard, but if he stays true to himself and his values, he will find the right way through. And contrary to his fear, this path of authentic, unapologetic leadership is less stressful and more fulfilling than he could have ever imagined.

Unapologetic leadership has transformed our lives. Through this book, I hope you'll discover the power it can have in yours.

Dr. Catherine Kyeremanteng, August, 2023.

Preface

My father, Solomon Kyeremanteng, was a man of many facets. Born in a quaint village in Ghana in 1939, he grew up amidst a large family. His pursuit of knowledge led him to Germany, where he completed his engineering degree. In 1967, he relocated to Edmonton and took on the role of managing Alberta's farm safety program. This role demanded his presence all over the province, leading safety talks.

During my childhood, I often accompanied my father on these provincial expeditions. We shared a lot of time on the road, marked by innumerable burger and fries pit-stops. These drives offered me a unique window into my father's world and his dynamic, funny, and charismatic personality. Solomon was well-known and loved by many; his charisma seemed to leave an indelible impression on everyone he met.

However, there existed a stark difference between the man the public knew and the man I knew at home. In private, my father could be stringent and demanding. A lesson that resonates with me till this day, fondly known as the First Rule of Solomon, states, "As a black person, you need to put in additional effort, outshine the white individual standing next to you. Be the clear choice so that when a decision is made, it inevitably falls in your favor. This way, regardless of the outcome, your conscience is clear. There's no room for regret." He'd often reinforce this idea, saying, "You gotta leave them no options."

I took my father's advice to heart, and it has guided me to where I am today. I'm now an ICU doctor and a palliative care specialist, the person who helps patients either recover their lives or transition from this world as comfortably as possible. Outside of medicine, I use my podcast -- Kwadcast -- among other platforms to advocate for change.

While medicine is my primary vocation, I've formulated four guidelines applicable beyond healthcare. They are equally effective within companies, political organizations, non-profits, sports teams, educational institutions, and social clubs. These principles are universal, underlining my unapologetic approach to leadership.

The Principles Of Unapologetic Leadership

1. **Fear threatens success. Values, not fear, guide effective decisions.**
2. **True leadership stems from those creating change. Favour action.**
3. **Outside-the-box thinking + action = Creative & Impactful Solutions**
4. **All progress must be rooted in equity and compassion.**

This book is dedicated to those ideals and the warriors who already practice them.

Unapologetically yours,

Kwadwo Kyeremanteng

Summer, 2023

Principle 1

Fear Threatens
Success.
Values, Not Fear,
Guide Effective
Decisions.

Wake Up Call in the ICU

It was 2010 and we had a young guy in our care who had a tracheostomy. It took him a long time to get off the ventilator. He was extremely reliant on chest physiotherapy that would help clear out his lungs. But there were financial cutbacks in the system and of course the first ones to go include physio and occupational therapists. It was a long weekend and there was no physio available to keep this patient going forward. As a result, he started having breathing problems again and his condition deteriorated so much he ended up back in ICU and back on the ventilator. All his progress was for nothing.

A week later a woman in her nineties came in from a nursing home with multiple medical problems including dementia. She ended up intubated and on a ventilator. She died. But because we didn't have access to family members and her medical history had gotten lost in the shuffle, we didn't know that her wishes were the opposite. She didn't want to be ventilated. $15,000 worth of interventions went into care she didn't even want.

When I witnessed what happened to those patients, I decided to take action. I started networking with colleagues who had the same frustration with the appalling amounts of waste and, ultimately, the less than optimal care we were giving people in general.

After obtaining a master's degree in health administration, in 2015 I founded the Resource Optimization Network (RON). Physicians, nurses, health economists, pharmacists, researchers and business academics were brought together to pool their knowledge with the focus on tangible ways of reducing spending and using existing resources wisely. All while not only maintaining but improving the quality of care provided to patients.

It seemed obvious to begin examining the most expensive forms of care first. I knew that would be the ICU. ICU is generally understood to consume about *20 percent* of a hospital's entire budget. On a Canada-wide scale, that translates to one percent of this country's entire gross domestic product. It costs three times more to maintain an ICU bed than a bed in a general ward.According to the Canadian Institute for Health Information (CIHI), the average stay in a hospital in 2021-2022 cost $7,619. Take into account the higher cost of an ICU bed and that an ICU patient can stay anywhere from four to fourteen days, depending on their condition and whether, frankly, they die or not.

Big bucks.

In one of our very first research projects, we looked at how much money it costs to admit patients more than 80 years old into the ICU. We found that the average length of stay is four days, with 35 percent of those patients dying. The average cost to accommodate an elderly patient varied from $31,679 to $65,857 depending on whether they returned to the ICU.

And here's the kicker – not everyone wanted that level of care, just as the woman I mentioned above didn't.

We have found that most patients and their families preferred comfort measures over life support. That, along with the high number of poor clinical outcomes, led us to conclude that for elderly patients the preference for comfort care reinforces the importance of discussions about palliative care as a way to not only to avoid undesired and potentially non-beneficial interventions, but to reduce costs.

Can We Always Afford "No Matter What"

We have to take the "no matter what" attitude out of the decision-making, from the bedside right on up to the board tables and political circles. A cultural mind shift is needed.

With a patient the question should be, can we help you achieve your goals? And if we don't think those gains are attainable, we need to present it in a way or explain it in a way to help a patient understand what is doable.

Now let's apply that kind of thinking to solving healthcare.

Rather than make a decision out of fear, let's make a decision that's going to work. We have to follow the data, look at the possibilities, and intervene with a decision that matters.

We have well-trained, intelligent dedicated people who can come together and work as a team to overcome serious challenges and get results. We have all the tools, all the toys at our fingertips. It's knowing when and how to use them to do what we are here to do: save lives and make people better.

Let me tell you what that looks like with yet another ICU scenario:

We had a patient come to us with COVID. He was in his forties and shouldn't have been high risk. Suddenly he was in need of more oxygen. His organs were failing, and we had to engage in a variety of interventions.

Our team came together and worked on his condition until, hours laters, he finally stabilized. We were cohesive, we were a unit, we were engaged. At the end of that day, I said to everyone: "We did good today, man."

That's what it's all about. Leaning into the whirlwind and working together so we can have the best possible outcome. We did everything the way it was supposed to be done to salvage that man's life. And it worked. That patient went home.

It's not like we don't have the means to make this health-care system work. We do. We have the expertise. We have the money. We have the desire to help. Let's sideline the fear and go unapologetically forward.

The Canary In The Coal Mine

Healthcare is, I believe, the canary in the coal mine of emerging workforce challenges. Volatility and carelessness result in the worst possible outcomes. In this business, the bottom line isn't profit or loss. The sick and dying don't care about that. With that in mind, I want my experiences and ideas to form a template that leaders and potential leaders in other fields can use and adapt to their own circumstances.

Healthcare in Canada, indeed, in many countries, is in such a deplorable post pandemic state, it's screaming for leadership and direction. Are you the one? You could be. I am telling my colleagues and others that no matter what part they play in the system, whether they are administrators, doctors, nurses or other healthcare providers that are experiencing all the crazy going on right now, everyone has the capacity to be the change if we dig deep enough. This challenge extends to leaders outside of healthcare as well. Are you in a think tank with concepts that can apply to healthcare? Bring it on. Suggest some changes, offer some start-up incentives. Let's do some idea exchanges.

The core of unapologetic leadership is exercising creative courage and inspiring it in others. It's finding the root of an issue and not being afraid to pursue avenues that aren't a quick fix. Where is the long game here?

We need to be brave in creating a work culture that allows these young, diverse minds to speak up without admonishment or threat of cancellation because they didn't know their place. Their energy, their willingness to buy into the long game isn't a resource we can afford to throw out. Retaining and nurturing your greatest resource – people – will allow them to see that if they speak out they will have an instant cohort of like minded unapologetic colleagues to support them.

We need to win this game, people. We need to pull together and put our differences behind us and focus. We need to end the myopic political gaze at the system and look in new directions. And those who have voices need to connect with those on the street who have never had a voice. We as moral, decent citizens have to reach those who are underserved by the status quo – racialized communities, the economically challenged, the disenfranchised – the folks who have taken all the hits, not just during COVID but throughout our country's history.

I'm not pretending to know all the answers. But I sure as hell am going to work toward getting them. We gotta listen to people out there and to each other. And by listening, we'll have a better chance of success. It takes teamwork, collaboration, and making decisions informed by data and not emotion.

This is just the beginning. We can talk about raising awareness, but we want to be that change. When we're unapologetic about our values, when we fuel our leadership with creative courage and collaboration, when we get our "juice" from morals, values and passion and not ego, we can provide solutions that will be sound, longterm, and efficient.

It's so easy to devote energy to limiting options, to say something is not possible. Of course it's possible.

Let's do the right thing and move unapologetically forward.

The Birth Of Kwadcast Nation

Going into the pandemic the Research Optimization Network had produced dozens of papers, all peer reviewed and published in medical journals. We looked at everything from the cost-effectiveness of palliative care to the overuse of antibiotics in ICU patients. Some of our work focused on very specific conditions and interventions.

We gathered a ton of info and made a ton of recommendations. So, who has read these papers? Who has implemented changes? What new policies were being put in place? Guidelines? Initiatives?

Who knows.

Despite these studies there was no tangible difference in how care was being delivered. Apparently collecting data and publishing it isn't enough. Now what? There are other papers out there that are more than 10 years old with recommendations and they're still not common practice even though they've shown effective methods for change.

We needed a way to take the information we had been gathering and put it out there so there could be action.

That meant knowledge translation: a way of turning information into real change by tweaking the way it's disseminated. Maybe we should be getting grants for pilot projects?

They may work, they may not. Someone's gotta start throwing spaghetti to see if it sticks to the wall.

I've never seen myself as a great speaker. But I liked the idea of challenging myself in a variety of formats. I can't say I've been very strategic about it, but I'm always in favour of action over just whining and bitching. I've done this my whole career. I always say be the change. Just do the right thing.

And that's when the idea of a podcast was born.

We needed to not only have the information, we needed to pitch it. In a perfect world if I could choose one group that had to notice what we're saying it would be those holding the purse strings because they ultimately have the ability to move the needle. Government officials, healthcare administrators, clinicians and fellow physicians, scientists, and others who can directly influence change are the ultimate audience, but I had to start the conversation somewhere. And I didn't want to leave out the grassroots. People in communities, living and working in the trenches – they needed to hear about the possibilities for change too.

In 2019 we began the *Solving Healthcare* podcast. The format features interviews and discussions on the topics of improving individual level health, improving healthcare delivery, personal experiences in healthcare, current events in the industry and new innovations.

We wanted each episode to be underpinned by the values of cost-effectiveness, dignity, and justice.

Sometimes it's just me talking from the front seat of my car about something that just happened that's awesome or maybe I'm ranting about an issue that's pissing me off. Or it could be a pre-planned zoom interview. Once I did a promo for a charity fundraiser while riding my bicycle. The Kwadcast has taken on a life of its own and I've had the opportunity to pair up with regular guests, do webinars, livecasts…anything that will get the message out there.

Right from the beginning the mission has been to challenge the status quo, explore gaps, assumptions, and different perspectives in the pursuit of finding solutions to problems in Canada's healthcare system.

In my very first podcast in September, 2019, I told my tiny audience that I wanted to keep it light, keep it real. I wanted to throw down. I wanted it to be a podcast that wasn't like reading from an academic journal boring the hell out of everyone. I wanted it to be clear so that people from any level of understanding could listen in and feel like change was not only possible but it was happening. I intended to give people a podcast that gave them hope.

My voice went out there with this jazzy intro music and man, I was feeling it. I was psyched. I was thinking, This is IT!

And then a couple of months later we were hit with the COVID pandemic.

We suddenly had to make decisions about the podcast's focus and decided that we would stay true to our original mission of searching out changemakers and exploring innovation, but now it was about what the hell was going on with the pandemic. We had the challenge of finding out the real information and to get it out there in a balanced, responsible way.

That was a hard pivot, especially when the media and the government seemed more interested in delivering scant statistics than using gathered data.

When the lockdowns were ongoing, there was no cost benefit analyses on how, say, indefinite school closures would affect mental health, physical concerns, and the overall effectiveness of our kids' immune systems.

We didn't factor in how that would affect the economy or the fate of our front line workers or the disruption involved in suddenly homeschooling our children around our jobs. No risk assessment was made, or at least none that came to light. If we had approached policy making from the very start with potential outcomes in mind for the entire public, we would not be in the crisis that we are in today, I assure you.

Because of my firsthand experience during that first wave in the ICU, I understood that the risk of COVID varied greatly among individuals. The elderly, individuals with metabolic health issues like diabetes and obesity, and those with weakened immune systems were particularly at risk. While we couldn't deny the gravity of COVID, it was also apparent that many in the population were at a lesser risk. The dominant sentiment was fear, amplified by media coverage and policy choices.

Cathy and I couldn't help but notice the looming mental and medical fallout from these overly specific decisions. The political nuances of the pandemic were hard to overlook. In our eyes, the overwhelming byproduct of the virus was fear. Considering our age, health background, and knowledge about the virus, it was evident to us that we, much like our kids and numerous others, were not in the high-risk category. The relentless lockdowns seemed excessive.

I recall saying to Cathy, "This wasn't what we were seeing. The prevalent fear being disseminated didn't match our deeper understanding of the situation."

Cathy, who is a psychologist, agreed. "If we keep this up, we're in trouble," she said.

And we made that conscious decision right there to speak out, to be the voice of reason. Even though it could jeopardize our livelihood, a calculated, compassionate message was too important not to share.

"Your family will always love you and support you, and that's all that really matters," Cathy said. We made that leap and geared the podcast toward exposing the dangers involved in maintaining a COVID-only focus. We had a micro-phone, we had an audience. They needed to hear a realistic, balanced message to counter the fear narrative. And that's how we operated.

The Human Toll

Look at your staff – what talent is there needing to be nurtured? What technological resources are on hand that are being ignored? What methods and modalities need to be kicked to the curb versus the ones that can be adapted for new challenges? Unapologetic Leadership means stepping outside your comfort zone, thinking outside of the proverbial box.

Your workforce already has, frankly.

They have been told to pivot so many times that they've become expert at it and they'll pivot their way right out of your organization if you can't meet their needs both now and in the future.

According to a report by the consulting firm Gartner, organizations are faced with historical challenges in engaging a sustainable workforce. The author, Emily Rose McRae, pointed out the need for finding and maintaining competitive talent will be different than in pre-pandemic times.

It ain't 2019 anymore, folks.

People are not only exhausted, but pandemic trauma will continue to linger. Organizations that don't address the needs of their workers' mental health and their workplace priorities will lose them to a place that will. Fostering skills and talent within existing staff will manifest new energy and drive. McRae says "stretch and upskilling opportunities for existing employees while meeting evolving organizational needs" is a way to not only maintain the headcount, but allows it to flourish in an otherwise jaded environment.

And let's not forget managers, especially middle managers. "The demands of today's working environment have left managers completely out of their depth. They feel pressure from above and below: they must implement corporate strategy with regard to hybrid work while also providing a sense of purpose, flexibility, and career opportunities." According to Gartner, providing fresh support and training to enhance managerial skills is vital.

In a nutshell, it means that old ideas are just that – old. Managers and leaders can either offer band aids or nourish encouragement – decision makers are facing no other option but to choose the best solution. It takes courage to choose it.

Yes, we are still in crisis mode, one that's evolved for all the reasons I've mentioned above. However, the time for knee jerk decision-making without front line input has passed. We are now in a shift and there is opportunity for those who are gutsy enough to seize it. Admittedly, for decision makers, especially politicians, that's a huge risk, because it could mean not getting elected again. Sustainable decisions in healthcare will likely mean deficit spending – it never looks good on paper and can be easily attacked as fiscally foolhardy. When you invest in prevention over prescription, you don't see instant results. It's an investment which will show itself worthy years from now. If it's going to take hold, now is the time to start laying down those necessary infrastructures.

Wouldn't it be refreshing if we could make our decisions based on our shared values instead of in reaction to potential blowback from someone trying to score election points .

Principle 2

True Leadership
Stems From Those
Creating Change.
Favour Action.

The Call To Lead

People are just *so* sick of the same old same old. I truly believe that if you want to be impactful, if you want to make a difference, adhere to your vision and reject fear.

Yeah, we're in trying times but we don't need thoughtless gestures. Quick fixes are akin to thoughts and prayers after a school shooting in the United States. No one wants the same cycle of crisis and token repair that ignores the root issue.

Straight up I'm telling you, if someone came to the microphone and said, look at this idea and let's work on it together, it would be received with crazy enthusiasm.

Who's around right now that anyone wants to emulate? Who can our kids look up to? If you want to be effective, you gotta be real. You have to throw out the cookie cutter and write the new recipe. It's time to quit placating to the polls or social media or whatever is driving popular opinion and get unapologetically inventive.

When I chat with someone who's stepping up, I get excited. Because they're bold. They're putting their voice out there and innovating, advocating, and manifesting what needs to be done in a broken system that relies way too much on tired and expired avenues for delivering services to a mentally and physically exhausted public.

15 Ways You Can Be An Unapologetic Leader

Now What?

So, you've decided that yep, I'm doin' it. I'm stepping up. I'm going to lead.

You can't do it all. You don't need to reinvent the wheel. You don't need to get stressed before you even start down this road. That's a recipe for burnout right there.

We've gone through why we need to take action. Here's the how.

1. Leave Your Ego At The Door. Stay Humble.

This ain't about you. No power tripping, no thinking you're going to be the answer to everyone's prayers. What you do need to take with you is courage, and to empower your team to have it as well.

2. Develop A Stomach For Difficult Decisions.

Take calculated risks, and stand up for what's right is vital if you're going to initiate any kind of change. Even if it's in the face of opposition or uncertainty, encourage other professionals to do the same. And remember, learn from your own mistakes and move on. Success comes from failure.

How do you find those people? Look around and see who's practicing your principles in their day to day work. Those are the people with the potential to join you in action.

You want to be a stakeholder in making the future of healthcare better? Then don't sit back. Courage means having the guts to not only bring forth new ideas but being willing to take charge of piloting them. Go beyond merely gathering evidence and data –use those as tools for your actions.

3. Focus On The Goal, Then Figure Out How.

Maybe you're struggling with a process that isn't working and you have an idea about what *can* work.

Remember, it's not about making your life better. It's about the people we're serving. This is the Why. Then it's about the What. What is it you want to achieve? What does your healthcare facility/organization need? What are your values?

Start with clearly defining and communicating objectives. If you've got a project that you think has teeth and want to make it actionable, do the homework and cost it out. Ultimately this is the absolute number one piece of information that policy makers want. Show how it will save money. If you can show decision makers the advantages in their own language, your concept is more digestible and it will move your vision forward off the paper and into reality. This is a key part of the How.

4. Break Down Your Objectives Into Manageable Achievable Goals.

Take what you want to accomplish and chop it up into attainable goals. My personal challenge is decision fatigue, so I tackle the hard stuff earlier in the day and leave the easier stuff until the afternoon.

I stack emails and answer them in sequence.

I define my tasks for the day and then focus on the one that will make the most difference. Increase your own efficiency so you can stay on task by biting off bits of your project a little at a time.

5. Listen, Truly Listen.

This is coming from a podcaster, the guy who goes on the media news panels and sits in the boardroom. I cannot say enough about the need to be transparent and open and to invite feedback. The worst thing you can create is an echo chamber where everyone just nods and agrees and then does nothing. That's just whining and bitching.

You want results. You want input. You want the options to flow.

It's up to you to create an atmosphere for a true exchange of ideas, where it's a discussion and not an argument. So when you walk in with that brilliant plan, make sure you've done the homework so you can answer the hard questions. And if you can't answer them, make sure you are open to working toward finding those answers.

6. Step Back When Disappointment Hits You In The Face.

Mike Tyson once famously said that it's fine to have a plan but it's what you do after you've been punched in the mouth that matters most.

If you've walked into a situation expecting all the love and you get criticized, step back a bit. Take a breath. Sit down with it for a couple of minutes and work through it.

I call it productive mode. I'll be sitting there feeling yucky and letting the self-talk walk through my brain, but that isn't going to help anyone. So quell that narrative and remind yourself, "I'm human. I'm doing all the good things. I'm going to use this moment to learn and move forward."

I can be my own worst critic and I know I'm not alone in that. If you're going to be transparent and open and focused, you have to accept what people say and *listen*.

Take what's been thrown at you, bad or good, and work through how that all fits into your goal. And then refocus on the goal with a more clear direction.

7. Ask The Doers.

If there was one aspect the COVID pandemic that felt most frustrating, it was not being empowered as health-care professionals. We felt like we had our hands tied by bureaucrats and politicians.

This can't happen anymore. Everyone loses when there is no balanced or informed policy making. Without empowerment, we'll just have a lot of talk and no action.

Let's talk about self-empowerment first, though. If you want to inspire others to take action, you have to believe that what you are doing will make a difference. And when you have that belief, you have to follow through. Put your values in action. Sitting on the sidelines is not acceptable when you have the means and there are people in need.

We who are in the trenches need more autonomy, so if you're in a position to demand it then do it. If you're in a position to offer it, do that.

Remember, you aren't going to have all the answers, but you can recognize the ability in others to help you find them.

8. Delegate, Delegate, Delegate.

Lean on your team. It brings them in and empowers them and leaves you the means to concentrate on your super-power, whatever that may be, and run with your gift wholeheartedly.

As a leader, you want to delegate so you don't get caught up in the minutiae. Put value on your own time and invest in a support staff that will allow you to be as efficient as possible

I hired my own research assistant in 2015. It was a game changer that allowed me to really invest in my strengths and launch my career. I went from producing one or two papers a year to ten.

By surrounding yourself with a team that can take care of all the details, you can invest more time into your own talents, become that much more efficient and give yourself a chance to grow. And here's a bonus: knowing your own bandwidth will help you avoid burnout. So recognize its worth and stay in it. Guard it.

9. Leadership Is Built On Accountability.

Take a close look at your own performance and your own results and then raise it up a few notches. If you are going to demand accountability from others, you have to know what that means in your own work. If there's a mistake, own up to it. If there's a win, acknowledge that. Being transparent about your contribution is key if you are expecting that level of service from others who may have what you need to see your vision through to fruition.

10. Don't Sit On The Sidelines.

If anyone is going to have any faith in your ability, you gotta be stellar in your own practices. This means knowing when *not* to delegate a task. You as a leader have to be willing to step into the dirty mess and navigate that. It keeps you humble and the ego in check. This is healthcare. It ain't no armchair traveling. If there's a crisis, it's literally life and death. In the ICU I can't stand at the door and let someone else take the fall if things go south. It isn't a discussion. Someone's life hangs in the balance. I have to be in it doing the best I can, relying on my team to work with me and not for me.

11. Bend.

Be ready to adapt and change course if a strategy is not working, especially in the face of rapidly changing circumstances. You applied for that grant and your pilot project is contingent on it. What if you don't get the money? Don't just drop your idea. Find another way to initiate it. Broaden your search parameters. Or you've got the grant and the project is going south. Recognize that the plan needs to go in a different direction.

Flexibility is about accepting compromises too, especially if the input you're receiving is coming from the folks on the ground who are actively engaged in the process.

Remember, being open to feedback will tell you if a strategy isn't panning out. This is the time to reassess and, with the help of your team, tweak and refine until a new course of action can be put into play. Then move forward.

12. Be Part Of The Team.

If you're in a management position, this is your chance to invest in your staff so you can provide opportunities for personal and professional development.

Healthcare professionals need to stay updated on new data, new procedures, new treatments, new approaches. If you can serve your staff with authentic opportunities for expanding knowledge and advancing their opportunities for career-building, they are more likely to stick around.

This is a top down thing, folks. Don't wait for someone to come and ask you for it. If you're in there observing your team at work, you're going to see where the needs and wants arise. Staying in touch with new information and offering professional development is not only great for retaining staff, it keeps everyone engaged in the ultimate task of doing the best for our patients.

Don't leave it up to them to figure this out for themselves. Discuss how to incorporate self-care into their daily lives. When our group developed *Solving Wellness* (read more about this on Page 44), we did it so it would speak specifically to healthcare providers and their needs because just saying "go to the gym" isn't good enough.

13. Exercise Your Empathy Muscles For The People You Serve.

Embracing empathy in your patient relationships will help you better understand how to treat them. What are their goals and desires? What input can family members offer in developing a plan that will help their loved one achieve this?

The work of healthcare providers is getting more and more harried all the time, but never be too busy to focus on the real stuff that matters. Let the patient and their families into your head and ensure that you've developed an atmosphere of authentic trust.

In the ICU that kind of empathy needs to be magnified by a thousand. And there's no reason why this can't apply to any other department in a healthcare facility or institution. Hey, it would be nice if politicians could take a page out of this, right?

14. Practice Institutional Non-Racism.

Here's an obvious one.

Encourage your organization or institution to really study how to bring more equity and diversity into their system. People with unique qualities can offer more insights that can expand and enrich healthcare. Recognizing those who demonstrate resilience and determination in the face of adversity can only help make the system more effective. This is life and death stuff, my friends.

15. Do NOT Succumb To Fear-Based Decision Making.

This is the BIG lesson I've learned from the pandemic: fear-based decisions suck. It's natural to make a decision based on fear as a response to some situations, but it can also be detrimental to our well-being and success. Fear can often lead to rash decisions that are not thought through and not aligned with your values and goals.

Remember that vision and purpose thing – what is the ultimate goal? Serving our patients. It's important to take a step back when faced with a crisis and reflect on the potential outcomes. Thinking through the options instead of just the worst case scenario can help you avoid making a rash decision with a narrowly focused outcome.

Consider how your decision aligns with your values and goals. Your choices will be more meaningful and fulfilling for both you and the people we're taking care of.

If you can't fully visualize all the options and scenarios, then ask for advice from trusted sources. Gather all the information you need to make an informed decision and weigh in with others on the possibilities.

Principle 3

Outside-the-box
Thinking + Action =
Creative &
Impactful Solutions

The First Rule Of Solomon.

As I mentioned in the preface, no one understood the obstacles facing black people better than my dad and he wasn't shy in telling me the antidote to that harsh reality.

"Leave them no excuses," he told me. "If two people are going to apply for the same position, you have to do more."

I remember bringing home an A average. "This isn't good enough," Dad would say. "You think they're going to hire you…or the Mark Campbells of the world? You need to do more. Leave people no other option but to choose you."

That principle holds for anyone advocating for change: the key is making a case so compelling that it would be obviously foolhardy not to act on it.

I often see a lack of critical thinking in healthcare. Both clinicians and politicians like to be right, so we stubbornly hang on to our previous methods and models because we're reluctant to change. We don't just need good listeners who are happy to just stay in their lane and work their way through the ranks, we need people who will take chances, stick their necks out and try something.

This is why I promote the idea of piloting projects on a small scale. Prove the concept in your own house from both health quality and financial standpoints. Then when you've got that data, amplify. The colossal amounts of waste in the system are a result of people trying to work with what they've got and not taking chances on new paths. It's time to unapologetically go forward with a new system.

Solving Wellness

We needed a forum to explore solutions as well as validate the feelings of isolation and loneliness ushered into our lives by the pandemic.

That's why, in 2021, we started our Solving Wellness online service.

Change management is at the core of this and every other endeavor we've taken on since putting together the Resource Optimization Network.

Here's what *Solving Wellness* looks like:

We've pulled together a group of physicians, researchers, psychologists, and wellness experts to provide online health and wellness content that is specifically geared toward healthcare providers. It's a collaborative process designed to help people make positive changes in all aspects of their lives.

When you join up, you'll discover a hub where you can find online expertise focusing on a wide variety of fields: medicine, psychology, mindfulness, yoga, epidemiology, and public and population health. We cover topics like nutrition, exercise physiology, sleep science, and relationships. It's a safe space for connection, for information, for advice.

People can sign up for a membership which costs only about ten bucks a month. We have about 500 members currently but it's growing and as we look to partner with organizations, I can see this scaling into a network of thousands.

Members have access to facilitated online peer support networks. There are discussion groups so people can feel supported and foster accountability to help with those steps toward taking control of their health and well-being.

There's a lot of content that could be anything from an online workout, live webinars, workshops and classes. We have e-books, podcast episodes, blog posts...everything designed so that members can fit this into their own schedule from home or wherever it's best for them to take this all in.

It's designed so people can regain a sense of control over their work and home lives. By doing that, they can gain the strength to stick their necks out and take action toward improving the system. If we're going to change this healthcare shitshow we've inherited, we need to have personal strength. That will translate to conviction, to making a difference.

One of the features offered is customized wellness for organizations. We work with the group at Bayshore Health-Care to provide workshops and retreats designed to improve employee health and wellness. This includes memberships to the online platform. It has been a truly rewarding experience seeing a fellow healthcare organization evolve and taking part in something that has been meaningful in reducing burnout.

Re-Energizing Professionals

Leveraging the use of personal support workers for patient care would allow nurses to be able to concentrate more on their skills. In a time when the system is bleeding from nurses quitting from burnout and job dissatisfaction, this small but vital pivot could re-energize a profession that, currently, few people want to join.

This topic was one of several inefficiencies discussed in a panel hosted by Adrienne Arsenault of CBC's The National in February, 2023 during the federal/provincial emergency healthcare summit. I was on that panel. Overwhelmingly, it was agreed by several of us that nurses and doctors need all the help they can get to do the jobs they signed up for and for care that patients deserve.

Alongside myself were a caregiver, a nurse who switched to a private clinic, a patient who was so fed up with surgery wait times he went to Lithuania for a knee replacement, and an economist who supports a total re-invigorating of the public system rather than relying on private services.

I took my message about prevention over prescription there, stressing that resources for maintaining both physical and mental health are needed desperately without these services being treated like they are luxuries. The economist, Armine Yalizyan, agreed. She believes that neglecting primary care results in more patients having multiple hospital visits. Everything from dental to mental care must be offered at no charge. Currently people have to pay separately for these services or they just can't afford it at all. People without means, she said, will end up with increasingly inferior care if more emphasis is put on private clinics to fill in the service gap.

"What's good for the individual is suicide for the system," she said. "We need to make the public system work better."

Centralized Wait Lists

Ms. Yanizyan was also adamant about a centralized waiting list for surgeries, along with dropping the provincial boundaries that limit the sharing of patient information. I heartily agreed with her assessment on both counts. People don't fully comprehend the level of costs we're talking about when it comes to system waste, I said. If a patient I'm seeing comes from a different jurisdiction, I don't have any of their chart details on hand. It means I can't see results from previous CT scans or other imaging, so it leaves me with no option but to order another one. It's so unnecessary and inefficient from a time standpoint as well which, for some patients, is literally a life and death issue.

In an article published in The Toronto Star soon after that panel discussion aired, Ms. Yanizyan pointed out that models for centralized wait lists and shared medical information have existed for decades but have never been initiated. Centralized wait lists deliver huge results. The practice helped the province of Saskatchewan.

More surgeries and shorter waits were possible by using existing facilities more intensively (more evenings and weekends). Staffing drew on more team-based care, encouraging people to work to the full scope of their competencies.

Surgical and post-surgical results were more clinically consistent, with fewer return visits to emergency.

Despite indisputable improvements, these initiatives never became a system priority. Why? Lack of focus? Reallocation of resources? New administrations with new political missions?

A centralized wait list pools referrals through a single entry point, triaged for urgency, and links to a booking system. It's one stop-shopping that requires co-ordination between booking systems and systems that track surgeries, on a daily basis.

I believe it would be more efficient in the long run to develop surgical hubs, that is, centres that are highly specialized and concentrate on only those types of surgery. Picture a knee surgery hub, one for hips, gallbladders, cataracts...they could operate like well-oiled machines. Perhaps a hub could be run like a business but funded with public dollars.

The Role of Private Clinics

The Ontario government is currently encouraging private surgical clinics to take up some of the waiting time slack. In Ms. Yanizyan's article that I referred to above, she is highly critical of this measure. She estimates that it is costing 30 percent more for those services and that the provincial government is dangling that financial carrot as a way of incentivizing clinics to get involved. She doesn't think it's an efficient use of taxpayer money.

I think the discussion about the role of private care is far more nuanced than that. Think of the amount of overtime that's being paid in the public system just to try and get the waiting lists rolling – some healthcare providers are getting paid double their rate because of increased overtime hours. You can't tell me that's better. Add to that, especially when it comes to acute care, the public system is considerably more inefficient. In a teaching hospital you can maybe get through four or five hips in a day whereas a private clinic can go through eight hip surgeries in a 24 hour period. They can narrow their focus and really hustle.

Engaging private clinics must be considered because, let's face it folks, we're in a crisis situation. We need to be mindful of our main goal, which is to get people healthy and heal them. If you're in your 60s waiting for a hip replacement and you can't do all the things that you love, those are some quality years that you're missing out on. To me, that's not okay.

Here's what I suggest: for clinicians and nurses defecting to private clinics, I think we need to limit private sector work to, say, 25 percent of their overall service. It would stem the talent drain significantly from the public system and deflate those waiting lists.

Let's keep in mind that healthier people living full lives will stay out of hospitals longer. It's all about balance.

Urgent Care

Along the same model of surgical hubs, I would like to see community urgent care clinics with a directed focus toward minor issues such as sprains, urinary tract infections...conditions that often send people to the Emergency Department. The ER wait times would be considerably alleviated with this kind of service which could be rolled out so that it could maintain a community focus so services could be tailored to the needs of a specific demographic being served.

Bringing More Foreign-Trained Doctors Into The System.

There are numerous barriers preventing foreign-trained doctors from being active in the workforce without having to retrain. Some doctors, yes, they aren't meeting Canadian standards, but for many they are needlessly directed into having to requalify. I know of a urologist who was foreign-trained, fully working and then came to Canada and has to do a residency all over again. Not three years, not two years, but five years. That's nonsense.

Sometimes language will be the barrier so in those cases, yes, more training would be necessary. However, we really need to examine how we can streamline medical English language training so that people who are almost capable can enter into the workforce quicker. People's abilities to work in Canada may be better than we think.

"Kwadcast Nation Listen Up."

We've been awarded a grant from the Ottawa Hospital and Montfort Research Institute to look at ways that we can help reverse metabolic disease in racialized communities!"

I was thrilled to make this announcement as a mini podcast episode in January, 2023. We got the green light for $90,000 to go into this project! Being sick isn't a race related issue – it's a marginalized community issue. It's a fact that a lot of people in Black communities are in less optimal socio-economic scenarios, living in multigenerational homes, and don't have the time or resources for high quality foods or hitting the gym. So, the project is designed to see what happens if we put together a multidisciplinary team that can leverage virtual health resources as a way of helping folks in these communities actually reverse disease.

Let's see what happens when we provide free access to a nutrition specialist, a health coach, fitness instructors, and an expert in diabetes.

Do you know how refreshing it is to have the opportunity to make hands-on changes for an underserved community? Chances like this don't come easily. It takes teamwork and it takes courage. And it means following the data. It's a logical course of action, right? An informed approach to preventative healthcare, one that can make people's lives better and ultimately, keep them away from me. Because no one wants to meet an ICU doctor.

It's all about prevention over prescription.

If we're going to have an effective system for delivering healthcare, we have to build on ways of keeping people from needing it in the first place. And that's why I was so thrilled to do that early January mini podcast. We identified a need, and now we get to take action.

"By no means am I saying this is guaranteed to be a success. You know, we've got to make sure it's feasible, we've got to make sure that our approach is something that's going to improve health and well being."

It's energizing to be part of a solution, so yeah, I was definitely humble bragging about our latest initiative:

I want to inspire those that are in the same spot. You guys reach out to me repeatedly. Other doctors. One who's close to the team told me, 'Enough! We're dealing with these patients at the late stages of chronic disease. I want to deal with them earlier. Let's get people healthy in general or if they already have metabolic syndrome, or poor health, then how can we reverse that? Let me prescribe the gym. Let me prescribe healthy foods. Let's inspire, let's be the change.

I want to reiterate this – the ideas and the way we execute them, they've got to come from the community. We can't just come in there and say, 'Hey, this is what it's gonna be'. We need to hear the voice of the community saying 'If you really want to see us make a difference it has to be front facing. It has to be within our leadership'. . . I'm not gonna pretend up front that I know all the answers, our group ain't gonna pretend up front that we know all the answers, but we are going to listen and by listening, we're going to have a better chance of success.

As I said in that excited mini-cast on my phone that day, it's just the beginning. We can talk about raising awareness, but we want to be that change.

Underlying Conditions

The pandemic gave we in the ICU some unique insight into what is making people sick. The majority of the extreme COVID cases that came to us were patients with underlying conditions – obesity, Type 2 diabetes, hypertension, and other cardiovascular risks. These are ALL conditions that can either be avoided altogether or reversed to a degree or completely eliminated.

There are huge medical, social and emotional costs from having a stay in the ICU. The residual trauma, depression and anxiety are enormous takeaways that continue to draw upon the healthcare system, not to mention the significant suffering for their caregivers and their families.

What are the interventions to help prevent an ICU admission?

I'll be the first to acknowledge that losing weight, getting fit and eating better is not an easy fix. It's one thing to state that lifestyle changes are needed. It's another to just leave it in the laps of the people who are affected by metabolic disorder. Remember at the very beginning of this book when I said we don't need more money to take care of people? Here's a prime example. We can change the focus of expenditures from merely treating disease to ushering in an era of promoting wellness as a primary part of our healthcare protocols. It makes so much sense, yet keeping people well is on the periphery of our overall care.

Why is that? Politically, the problem is that you're not going to see that investment pay off for years. That bottom line result isn't instantaneous. It isn't sexy enough for political gain. So ideas and initiatives that are going to gain traction are going to be ones with proven results. This is what we hope to achieve with the pilot project.

I started talking about simple wellness initiatives on social media during the pandemic as a preventative way of reducing hospitalization and death from COVID. Yes, the vaccines were amazing as a quick and needed response to a crisis, but what about the next time? I would argue that we are actually in the midst of the next time with the overwhelming wait times for emergency care and surgeries.

When I began this discussion, people responded positively to it. I used myself as an example about how I incorporate wellness initiatives into my day to day life. I wanted people to know that how we treat our bodies daily has a compound impact on our health over time. And I wanted then, and now, to empower people to change.

It's Not A Level Playing Field

Since those early podcasts, I've incorporated more and more emphasis on prevention as a course of action that we should all have access to. It needs to be acknowledged that there is no level playing field for wellness. Limited income and lack of transportation can mean that many Canadians are too isolated to go to the gym or eat the right foods. And with the added volatility of inflation, that accessibility window is beginning to close even more.

We can reverse a lot of what's hurting our health if we share the right information and access the right tools. It doesn't have to be expensive or rigid. Improving metabolic health means investing in ways to let people have access to higher quality foods. It means making our cities more walkable. It means promoting healthy living in culturally appropriate ways.

What if we take collective action and support discount rebates for gyms? What about subsidizing high quality food? Let's think about ways that we can reach out, educate, and reach those that are at highest risk. Honestly, investing in prevention has such huge compounding effects and could be generational.

Imagine if we could take the cost savings of preventing someone from entering the ICU and reinvest it into wellness initiatives. Instead of spending $50,000 (which was the cost of a single COVID ICU patient) to treat a person for preventable conditions, imagine what you could do in a community with that kind of money. Imagine having a neighborhood health coach or bringing gym equipment to a person's house who needs it. A couple of thousand bucks invested in a simple solution like that would mean an entire household could have access to the equipment. There are solutions there if we just start that out of box thinking instead of approaching treatments in the same traditional ways.

If your neighbor is a Type 2 diabetic, the amount of resources that they're going to use in their future years is tremendous. The medication, the admissions to hospital, the scanners…the amount of money that we spend to take care of those patients is insane. A reversal of their condition would mean fewer hospital visits, less medication, a longer lifespan, and a decreased likelihood of landing in ICU…it's just a matter of prioritizing it. Personally, I get inspired when I see a loved one's health journey become contagious. You can see the ripple effect when a neighbor shouts out and says, "Hey Charles, I hear you came off your diabetic meds. How did you do that?" Then Charles becomes a champion, the go-to guy for information, and his success becomes amplified and helps the next person.

While politicians may like to brag about instant outcomes, the real solution involves investing our energies and resources into the process. Think about it from a completely personal level. Oh, you got outside three times this week? That's a win right there. That's the brag material, not that you lost five pounds. Celebrating the forming of healthy habits, the action and not the results is where the success really is. So if we're going to truly get a payoff with the public health bucks we spend, then it involves having faith in the long term. Instead of the crash diet, let's focus on proceeding in a way that turns regular, good habits into lifegiving ones.

Mental Health Suffering

One of the other offshoots of a scaled wellness initiative will absolutely be improved mental health. It's a part of the human condition and yet psychological help is treated like a luxury item. The pandemic left many of us in a more precarious mental health state. People suffered from social isolation, depression, anxiety, bullying and even eating disorders. Kids in particular have suffered, I believe, and it's imperative that we get resources and tools to help with their recovery. Childhood is where we lay the foundation for healthy habits, yet the pandemic has interrupted their mental development to extremes. And it's even worse in communities that were already challenged with economic or racialized stressors.

Because COVID protocols didn't balance the harms of the virus with the harms of the mitigation measures, we are left with a generation of young people who had to go for years without having access to their friends, extended family, mentors and other social outlets. That takes a toll.

If there is anything that ignites within me the need for leadership in healthcare, it's our youth. They need examples of good leaders and they need to be the core reason for promoting wellness. Here in Ontario, I feel that the way the pandemic was handled was the antithesis of what leadership should be. That there weren't student uprisings against the fear-based mandates that were put in place worries me. Youth have lost their mojo. When universities were mandating three vaccine doses before getting students to even walk onto the campus, there was very little impetus in questioning these rules, even though they ignored data collected about myocarditis in highly vaccinated youth.

When virtual classes became a norm and there was no student revolt, well, that just scared me. As 18 to 22 year olds in my time, we didn't need a big reason to create an uproar. It could be something as small as wanting to double the on-campus parking fees. So yeah, I worry about our youth. A lot.

I used to think they needed all the help they could get to find their sense of authority and agency.

As it turns out, maybe they are. The catch is it's in ways that traditional management and decision making couldn't anticipate.

An Ounce Of Prevention

Dr. Lucy McBride, a regular podcast colleague of mine, often states that health is not just the absence of disease. She believes we are in a mental health emergency as a result of pandemic lockdowns and school closures. There has been "unmeasurable suffering from a loss of normalcy", she says, and that children took the brunt of it.

As the data came out during 2021 and 2022, there was no doubt that children were being impacted more than any other demographic. And as we found with COVID stats in general, the worst areas of suffering occurred in racialized communities. It wasn't just the learning loss that affected children and youth, it was overall health. The unintended consequence of lockdowns is that the people who needed the most help got the least of it. Now is when we need to offer more focus to those who are still suffering from the consequences.

This is a watershed moment that's not only imminent in healthcare, but for any organization in any field. The echo of all that isolation means that emerging employees are coming into the workforce compromised from pandemic trauma. Remember the Gartner report I referred to at the beginning of this book? One of the future work trends identified by their research is the need for work environments to take stock of this and incorporate wellness into their organization's culture.

From the report: "Most humans, and that includes current and incoming employees, are still experiencing pervasive mental health challenges as a result of the societal, economic and political turbulence of recent times. This may decrease productivity and performance, as well as increase angry outbursts, no-notice quitting, workplace conflict and sudden underperformance."

A survey Gartner conducted showed that a whopping 82 percent of employees desired that their organization see them as a whole person rather than just a worker.

The report specifically refers to Gen Z – this cohort's pursuit of educational and career goals were adversely affected by pandemic isolation, not to mention missing out on "soft skills" such as negotiating, networking, speaking confidently to an audience, and maintaining social stamina and attentiveness.

Recommendations include:

- Proactive rest to help employees maintain their emotional resilience and performance, rather than offering rest as a recovery solution after both have plummeted. It could look like offering personal days before high demand work period as well as allotted wellness time;
- Discussion opportunities to work through challenges and difficult topics without judgment or consequences;
- On-site trauma counseling, while training and coaching managers on workplace conflict and holding difficult conversations with employees

In addition to the above, the Gartner report also recommends increasing workplace support for diversity and inclusion even though there may be pushback from existing employees. This is coupled with the trend of employees charting nonlinear paths for themselves, for example, applying for jobs outside of their current area of expertise. Managers will need to be mindful of the widening girth of non-traditional sourcing methods and candidate pools, not to mention having to pull back from concerns about industry experience and technical skills.

Students and new hires have had to do their share of pivoting during workforce and academic upheavals in recent years. Now they are becoming unapologetically resourceful about taking back control of their lives. It's not up to them to do the adapting. It's up to organizations to welcome this challenge and channel all that energy by meeting their needs and fostering new ways of maintaining their loyalty. Strong leaders who recognize this energy shift will find ways of celebrating it rather than balking at it.

Principle 4

All Progress Must
Be Rooted
In Equity And
Compassion

Every Second, Every Minute, Every Day

As a black person in healthcare, I have found that some of my viewpoints come across as radical and counter to our goals of keeping people well. The lack of diversity in the board-room has resulted in the highest needs of marginalized people ignored or unnecessarily delayed.

I have participated in a few policy discussions with influential people within Ottawa and the province, giving a voice for those members of the population who have never been represented at the table. As the pandemic wore on, the idea of keeping schools closed resurfaced periodically. I argued against it.

As the data rolled in after that initial period of unfamiliarity with COVID, it was becoming clear that school age children were not at high risk. Keeping schools closed wasn't a balanced or informed decision. I pressed hard to keep schools open because I was – and still am – concerned for the mental health of racialized and economically marginalized kids. We needed to weigh the moral cost of a policy and consider the more nuanced ramifications before slapping out another blanket directive.

Underprivileged kids may not have a home situation where on-line learning is even an option. They may not have a computer or the internet. They may not have a parent who can afford to stay home with them or be in a work from home scenario.

In Ontario, the government had been advocating for more lockdowns with the wrong parameters informing their decisions – what are the unions going to say? How is that going to be received with voters? Most decision makers were too old to have school age children or too privileged to realize that, for some children, school is going to be the only outlet in their lives where they can be mentored. For some kids, a coach or a teacher may be the only role model they have. Taking that outlet away would undermine their mental and physical health. If and when those members of our population suffer, it would inevitably result in more illness in the future.

This is why these core decision-making bodies need diversity. It gives an alternative, more inclusive, and expanded perspective in a place where otherwise everyone looks the same with similar experience and backgrounds.

These folks who could just get their food delivered or order their supplies online – they didn't look like the ones who were delivering that food or packing those orders. Those people looked like me. Their values didn't include the essential workers who were out there with more exposure to the virus. Their comfort zone was their only perspective and when everyone else has the same point of view, decisions are made in a vacuum.

When there was discussion about mandating COVID vaccinations for students, I spoke out against that too. Again, having a racialized perspective allowed me to argue that not everyone is going to buy into that policy, for so many reasons. Public health policies have not been kind to Black and Indigenous peoples. There is an underlying sense of mistrust of the system that has weaponized "health" to exploit or harm these folks. Getting these populations engaged in a vaccine drive isn't just a given.

The hesitation to participate is culturally ingrained. If we are to achieve better results we need to acknowledge and address that reluctance.

Here are a couple of grim examples of healthcare mistrust from racialized communities – some of it alarmingly recent:

The Tuskegee Effect – Over Their Dead Bodies

In 1972, the New York Times broke a story about syphilis victims that were left untreated for 40 years in the name of medical research at the Tuskegee Institute in Macon, Alabama.

It was revealed that a cohort of American Black men were serving as human guinea pigs, going without medical treatment for the disease even though penicillin had been found to be an effective therapy about 10 years after the study began.

The story revealed that the men were promised free transportation to hospitals, free lunches, free medicine for diseases other than syphilis and free burial after autopsies were performed. In 1969 a study of 276 untreated men showed that seven had died as a direct result of the disease. Of the 400 men in the original study group, 154 died of heart disease.

When the paper published details of the Tuskegee experiment in 1972, only 74 of the original test subjects were still alive, with 128 having died from the infection or complications. Forty of their wives had been infected, and 19 children were found to have congenital syphilis.

No one was ever prosecuted for their role in the deaths of 399 men.

Ignored To Death

Indigenous peoples in Canada have borne a disturbing brunt of racist policies and inaction, resulting in lower health outcomes than anyone else in the country. The majority of people who die in waiting rooms are Indigenous.

Vile stereotypes are at the root of a variety of negative health impacts: stress arising from perceived discrimination, denial of access to resources that actually fit peoples' needs, internalized stigma, and the stress and tense social interactions that arise from anticipated negative treatment.

Aboriginal men have a lower life expectancy – 70.3 years versus the average of 79 years for other Canadian men. The same goes for women in this group – 77 years compared to 83 years. Infant mortality rates are higher too – in Manitoba the rate is almost double the national average

In September, 2008 an aboriginal man named Brian Sinclair was in Winnipeg. First he sought care from a family physician at a primary care clinic, and then was sent by taxi to the Health Sciences Centre a few blocks away. He entered the emergency there in a wheelchair where he spent the next 34 hours waiting to be attended to. He died. From an easily treatable condition. In Manitoba's most comprehensive health-care facility.

Video footage reviewed in an inquest five years later revealed that nurses would just walk right by Brian.

In 2020, 37 year old Joyce Echaquan died at a hospital in Joliette, Quebec. Her own Facebook video footage showed staff mocking her as she lay suffering from stomach pains. She was called stupid, harassed for making too much noise, and told that she was in withdrawal from illicit drug use. Unattended, she died from pulmonary edema, a type of respiratory failure.

Covid Impacts On Racialized Communities

It became evident as the pandemic wore on that race matters in terms of health outcomes.

In February, 2021, Canada's Chief Public Health Officer Dr. Theresa Tam released a report on the impact of COVID on racialized communities. In Ottawa and Toronto, she noted that these populations experienced anywhere from 1.5 to five times more cases than non-racialized populations. And First Nations people living on reserves had up to 69 percent higher rates of infection.

Here's what Dr. Tam had to say: "These disproportionate impacts among racialized and Indigenous communities are not due to biological differences between groups or populations. Rather, they reflect existing health inequities that are strongly influenced by a specific set of social and economic factors – things like income, education, employment and housing that shape an individual's place in society . . . Members of racialized communities are more likely to experience inequitable living and working conditions that make them more susceptible to COVID, such as lower incomes, precarious employment, overcrowded housing, and limited access to health and social services. Many face increased risk of exposure to COVID due to their employment in front-line essential occupations with frequent contact with other people and a limited ability to work from home."

These "historical inequities" have existed in systems and institutions over many generations, she noted. "This continued generational systemic racism and mistreatment within the health system has led to considerable wariness within racialized communities, and **a significant lack of trust in these systems and institutions**. This lack of trust has contributed significant COVID vaccine hesitancy among the Black and Indigenous, as well as other racialized communities," Dr. Tam concluded.

Here are some bleak numbers to back up these claims. This is from a StatsCan report released in August, 2022 which analyzed COVID deaths in Black, South-Asian and Chinese communities:

Overall, the COVID mortality rate was significantly higher for racialized populations (31 deaths per 100,000 population) compared to the non-racialized and non-Indigenous population (22 deaths per 100,000 population).

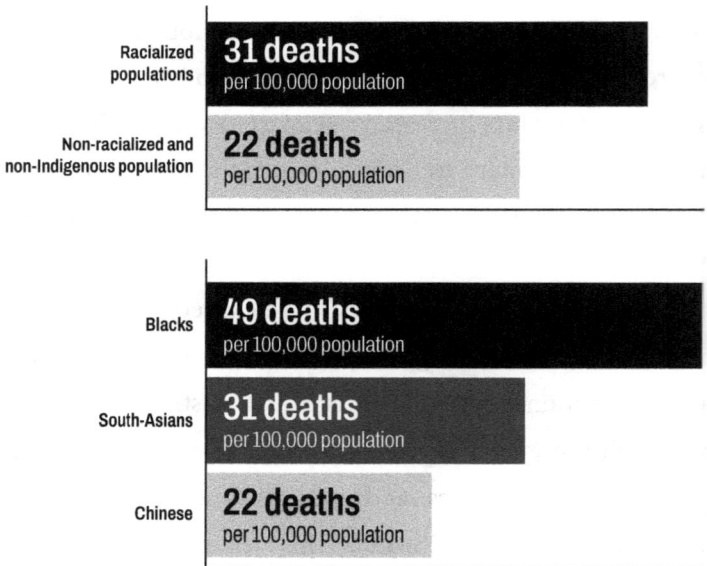

Racialized populations	**31 deaths** per 100,000 population
Non-racialized and non-Indigenous population	**22 deaths** per 100,000 population

Blacks	**49 deaths** per 100,000 population
South-Asians	**31 deaths** per 100,000 population
Chinese	**22 deaths** per 100,000 population

The mortality rate ratio between Black people and the non-racialized and non-Indigenous population was more than two times higher – 2.2 times.

"Within the total Canadian population, males had 1.6 times higher age-standardized COVID mortality rates than females. Among the male population, Black males had the highest COVID mortality rate (62 deaths per 100,000 population), followed by South Asian males and Chinese males. A similar pattern was observed among females. Among the female population, Black females had the highest rate of mortality (41 deaths per 100,000 population) followed by South Asian females. Chinese females had the lowest mortality rate (16 deaths per 100,000 population)."

The report noted the same parameters that contributed to these deaths as indicated by Dr. Tam in her report – housing, low income, and historic racism.

"Black people had the highest difference of COVID mortality risk between those not living in low income and those living in high income . . . the mortality rates were almost three times higher compared to Black people not living in low income and 3.5 times higher compared to the non-racialized and non-Indigenous populations living in low income."

The report also goes on to say that research suggests that Black people "tend to experience poor quality preventative healthcare in early life which contributes to the development of chronic health conditions in later years that can increase the risk of death due to COVID.

Unapologetically Black

"I'm given all these opportunities, which I should be grateful for but...our ICU research group ..we are one of the most prolific producers of papers globally in critical care. And several of these conferences we've said, hey you guys want to talk to us about cost, resource utilizations, end of life care..whatever, we've got tons of papers. No one rings at the door. But the BLM hashtag blows up and NOW you wanna come and talk to us about racism in healthcare and all this shit and I'm like, c'mon y'all. You wanna talk about this? Look at the body of work we're producing and NOW you're calling?"

Me – a podcast moment ranting about black trauma being suddenly cool

Honestly, if you told me that I would never have to give one of those racism talks again, I'd be fine.

Standing in front of 200 white people telling them why racism sucks? I don't love that.

It just stirs up so much emotion. I have to stand there and open up. It's like, boom, and I instantly feel it when I am looking at a crowd and I'm talking about my dad telling me that you have to leave them no options, that you have to do more. Because you're black. And then thinking about George Floyd, suffocated to death in plain sight. Nope, I don't like it.

It's not that I fear it. It's…uncomfortable, y'know? It means having to be vulnerable. It means having to relive all the crap I've put up with my whole life that isn't going *away*. And since the Black Lives Matter movement began focusing on systemic racism, it means being the token diversity spokesperson in whatever building I happen to be working in at the time. Just picture white folks sitting around the table scanning for someone and then it's "Oh yeah, Dr. K would know about that stuff" and suddenly I'm the expert on the subject.

But opening up means forming connections. It can create some real engagement with your crowd. And yeah, you see it. So as much as I don't like being publicly vulnerable, I have to remind myself of the value of doing something that will be a catalyst for the greater good.

Being a black doctor means being an anomaly. It means having a patient notice you in the hallway and get excited because there's someone on the team who actually looks like them. It means having people ask if you're a "real" doctor. It means being the only black kid in a med school class of 130 students and people wondering if you got some special treatment to get there.

Being an outspoken black critical care doctor in a hospital is one thing. Being the only six year old black kid on a hockey team is where I learned that I was different. That experience was my first real lesson in racism.

As kids, we were outside constantly. There wasn't anything I didn't play. Football, soccer, basketball, volleyball...but hockey was my number one sport. We played a lot of street hockey as well as being on a team.

It was the 80s and 90s and it was Edmonton, not the most diverse place in the world, right? And here I am, the black kid whose parents were from Ghana. I became aware very early on that I was different. Yeah, I was called names. It started when I was about four years old. A lot of racial slurs. That part was...hard.

My parents' philosophy was that it was best to ignore it, not let anyone see you flinch. If they see that it's not having an impact they'll let up. I mean, once in a while they'd get the teachers or the school administration involved. But for the most part I learned to take it and to hide my feelings about it.

Hockey, though, that was a different scenario because nobody really policed that.

I remember once playing in North Battleford, Saskatchewan. I was our only black player. My growth spurt came late, so I wasn't a big kid and I remember just being scared for my life. Every second player had something they'd call out – "Go back to Africa". "Monkey". And of course, the N-word. But it was more than that. Hockey's a violent sport. They were literally telling me they were going to kill me. I wasn't even thinking about the game. It was about survival. I don't remember in detail, but no one else was being told they were going to get killed.

But I never let them see me scared. And that's how I rolled until I was older and bigger. When I began to defend myself the slurs and the threats became less common.

But the racism never stops. It just becomes more veiled.

My life is filled with microaggressions. "Oh man, you're pretty articulate." "You speak surprisingly well for a ..." They won't say it, but what they mean is "black guy". Or this: people who alter their speech when they speak to you. "What's up, brother? What's up, my homie?" Ugh.

You get used to what you know and you act accordingly. You know when you're the only black person in a classroom and you're going to draw a lot of attention because you're different. I can walk into an elevator and if there's a white person in there I have to make a point of not standing too close so I don't seem threatening.

As a young adult hanging out at the West Edmonton Mall, it may have looked like I was having fun but the whole time there would be this running commentary in the back of my mind. I resisted going into stores because the questions would come: "Are you shopping? Are you planning on buying anything?" It's exhausting.

And then there are the not so micro aggressions.

I remember being 23 years old and driving home late one night. It was about 12:30 and the sirens went on behind me.

And I was alone in my car. Sadly, I've seen how aggressive the police can be and I know people who have been assaulted. So I was nervous…no, I was scared to my core. So I just took the phone and called Cathy. We were still dating back then. And I told her, "Just stand by, I don't know what's going on." And then the police talked to me and said something about a tail light. To be honest, I can't remember much about the conversation. I just remember it being scary because it was night and we were in a quiet area. If it was daytime I wouldn't have thought twice about it but alone in the dark like that, well, it could have really gone south.

Another time we got pulled over in Michigan and I had left my wallet in the trunk, so I was forced to be the one getting out of the car. Because this was Michigan, I felt the need to be ultra cautious in terms of how I was physically retrieving my wallet. I was certain to avoid any sudden movements and to articulate what my next steps were going to be. I wasn't going to get shot in Michigan.

These incidents ran like a b-roll in my head when I was part of a session on "Diverse Voices" at the 16th annual National Pharmaceutical Congress in November, 2022. I delivered a keynote address and brought up George Floyd's murder in May of 2020. That very public slow death ignited the BLM movement and with it the scrambling of hundreds of organizations to claim they were anti-racist and pro-diversity, terms that don't really mean anything without action to create fundamental systemic changes.

"I don't know how many people have watched the full nine minutes of this event. I've got to tell you there's nothing so viscerally difficult and hurtful to see than a grown man treated worse than an animal. A grown man was asking for his mom, and in broad daylight, was allowed to die. As a black individual, this takes you back to all the previous incidents of police violence. You can't help thinking about your own experiences when you've encountered racism ... In medical school, I was asked if there was an affirmative action or a quota and why I was in the building. And even recently when I was introduced as chief of the department, a patient was questioning, saying "chief of what department?" Like that's not possible."

Turns out living with racism has given me some skills that lend themselves to good leadership, though if someone told me this when I was a kid I would have given anything to not have it. I spent a lot of time wishing I wasn't black or that I had a different name.

The F*#k You Co-Efficient And Other Leadership Lessons For The BIPOC Community

1. Do More And If Necessary, Do It Angrily.

You think I can't do something? You think I won't be qualified? I always make sure I have more than what I need to prove my credentials.

It means creating a portfolio, a resume where there is evidence of so much good work that an institution can't not have you at the table. I leave them no other option. Oh, my colleague has written five papers this year? I'm going to do 20. They did 10 weeks of clinical time? I'll do 15.

Get angry. Own it. I want you to tell me I can't do something. I want you to tell me that this research program is going to fail. I want you to tell me that I could never be the head of an ICU department. I want you to tell me this podcast won't get anywhere, then at the end of the day I can say, "F*#k you. I told you so."

I call this the F*#k You Coefficient. As a person of colour, you could be that advocate that is sitting at the table offering alternative, expanded viewpoints on the effectiveness of decisions that could have a direct impact on the lives of individuals in racialized communities.

2. Monetizing Your Expertise.

First and foremost, I want to stress that your racialized experience is worth something. I mean financially.

If you as a BIPOC healthcare provider are being approached to speak about your experiences at a conference or as a media spokesperson, that's some valid expertise you're offering.

Canadian healthcare is predominantly populated with white people. You have a specialty focus that you can bring into the mix and you owe it to yourself to recognize that and to make your peers recognize it too.

If someone is asking for our unique point of view and it is triggering racist trauma, you need to be compensated for that. No compromise.

3. Think About The Next Person.

Being on the receiving end of racism sucks, right? And it can really piss you off, but you have to take that anger and channel it into something positive. What solutions can you bring to the table to lessen the chance of what happened to you happening to someone else? How can you make it better? Focus on the opportunity to change that boogie. You deserve not to have that trauma taking up space in your head without some sort of payoff. How can you make it better for others?

4. Lean Into Obstacles.

No one likes to acknowledge an experience that leaves them feeling vulnerable or trying to navigate a system that's stacked against you right out of the gate. Examine what it is that's holding you back and then work through that stuff.

5. Be Open To New Avenues Of Support.

When Dr. Onye Nnorom was talking on the Kwadcast about Afrocentric vaccine clinics during the pandemic, she told me that black community leaders had to seek advice from Indigenous communities about how to do it (See page 99 for more insight on Dr. O). They had experience navigating all the government levels for setting up healing centres for their people that provide culturally appropriate services in a safe environment. That input allowed black urban clinics to not only open quicker and more efficiently, they had a model for serving their communities more effectively.

6. Seek Out Other Leaders.

Share your knowledge and experiences with other BIPOC leaders. It not only reinforces your own vision and gives you "the juice" to recharge your batteries, it's a great way to compare notes. What works? What ideas do others have for advocacy or specialized services?

And don't just limit your scope to your own age group. There are a ton of young people with freshly charged energy coming into healthcare who can offer insights and approaches that those of us in more established careers may not have considered. Developing a camaraderie with other leaders can only serve to expand our collective horizons.

7. Be Generous With Your Time.

This is related to seeking out other leaders and maybe even mentorship, but if you've got a particular insight or experience that someone else needs, be generous with your time and offer them support, advice, networking possibilities or whatever it is that can give them a better edge. As racialized healthcare providers, we need to be positive and transparent about that. Maybe it's an opportunity to pay if forward, but being that reliable source for someone else helps us all as a whole.

8. Consider Mentorship.

One of the challenges for BIPOC healthcare professionals is that the system was built for the needs of white people. Our institutions and organizations have built in systemic racism that creates an imbalance for opportunities. If you see an individual or a group of individuals who need guidance in navigating this system, offer it.

Those with established careers have seen the obstacles and the challenges, developed networks and know the ropes. Most young people from racialized communities don't come with a comfort zone. Chances are they don't have a family tradition of going into medicine and have no connections or peers to help them along in building their careers. Change up the narrative for them and turn "I can't" into "I will".

9. Get A Seat At The Table.

One of the most impactful ways of making change is to get a set at the table. You've worked hard, applied the F*#k You Coefficient, and now you're in a position to be offered a key position where your input on decisions will have direct effects.

10. Go For It.

This is your moment to really show that you have some creative solutions to offer. Your different and unique perspective WILL be new to the room, I assure you. When there is at least one person of colour at that table, that is a point of view that has never been heard before. You can offer proposals that creatively address issues of diversity and inclusion as well as possible solutions for longstanding challenges.

This is the opportunity to steer the narrative about racialized communities into a different direction. Instead of communities being a problem, you can highlight how they can be the solution. Call it Ubuntu or whatever you want but this is IT.

My Unapologetic Hall Of Fame

As a sports lover, I am a big fan of Halls of Fame, hockey, football, baseball, you name it.

My Hall of Fame is filled with the unapologetically great people I know and work with - many of them on the Kwadcast - who embody the principles of unapologetic leadership. This list is by no means complete, in fact I look forward to adding many more, very soon.

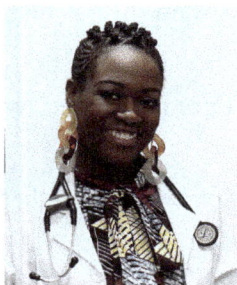

Unapologetically Inclusive

Dr. Onye Nnorom

Sometimes being racialized delivers the ultimate good, especially when it's in the trenches.

Dr. Onye Nnorom finds her advocacy is most effective at the street level, specifically in black and racialized urban areas of Toronto. A family doctor, past president of the Black Physicians' Association of Ontario (BPAO), and a public health specialist, "Dr. O" got her street cred working as the lead for the chronic disease prevention team at TAIBU Community Health Centre in Scarborough, a health centre specifically geared towards black people.

When we spoke it was 2021 during the midst of the pandemic. We got real about the need for community-based healthcare initiatives, traumatic racism, and the need for a system wide "renaissance" where equality and diversity are more than just buzzwords.

It was one of those occasions where I got re-charged for advocacy work.

At that time there was enough data available to show that Black people were unequivocally the hardest hit by COVID, even though the prevailing attitude had been that this virus was going to be "the great equalizer", meaning everyone from all demographics were going to be vulnerable. It wasn't, though. Black people comprise a large portion of the Toronto area's essential workers who don't get paid sick days, use public transportation, live in densely populated households and, Dr. O pointed out, have already compromised immune systems from the stress of systemic racism.

That race-based data wasn't originally in the game plan, but the BPAO advocated hard for it because, predictably, it ended up showing what people already knew would happen.

"The system is predisposing us to disease," said Dr. O. Because so many BlPOC healthcare voices are not getting places at the table, it meant that communities themselves had to rally to get vaccine hesitant people into clinics for information that would convince them that this particular public health initiative wasn't going to hurt them.

Dr. O described clinics where music would be playing, food offered, and community leaders and volunteers would gather to invite people in for a discussion – vaccines were suggested as a way of celebrating community wellness. Personal action as a contribution – empowering people through bodily agency – changed the narrative from a negative to a positive.

Unapologetically respecting the patient. This is how it should be all the time, not just in times of crisis.

Dr. O and I agreed that when health policies are being considered, they must be from a point of view of equity and diversity. Decision makers must use racial impact assessment tools along with health equity assessments to draw the lens away from the dominant culture ie. white people. Broadening the field of input and data can only better inform future directions. Ultimately, it would lead to wellness and reducing the amount of illness in racialized communities overall.

Doctors take an oath to do no harm. More emphasis using widened parameters will in time generate more trust in the healthcare system and allow all people to feel their lives are valued. Because, as Dr. O pointed out, during the pandemic when tragedy struck and a family member ended up dying alone, BIPOC folks had that extra fear – is it because of racism?

That's a heavy weight to bear.

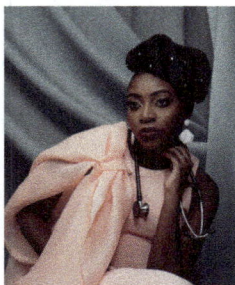

Photo credit: Christie Vuong

Unapologetically Activist

Dr. Chika Oriuwa

"Code Blue and the deep hues of my skin remind me that this is more like Code Black – meaning that there's an imminent threat. Suspicious object on hospital grounds."

From her spoken word poem, "Woman, Black"

When Chika Oriuwa gave the valedictory address to her University of Toronto graduating class in 2020, she was the only black person out of 259 medical students. The ONLY one.

Our podcast chat was a game changer for me. This woman's advocacy for Black students has turned her into a warrior, a goddamned HERO.

I identified so much with what she told me – the questions about her credentials which led to imposter syndrome creeping in, feeling isolated, having to weigh whether to speak up about obvious systemic racism. "Do I engage or educate?" Because speaking up could mean possibly jeopardizing future opportunities or being labeled a troublemaker. The constant risk assessment of taking action or letting it go.

She talked about how she and some fellow Asian classmates once went on a shopping trip to New York and were being questioned by an American border patrol guard. Once it was determined they were all students preparing for medical school, the guard focused on Chika and said, "Even you?" as if that was somehow impossible for a black woman.

We talked about how, when a black kid suggests they'd like to go into medicine there is such an overwhelming sense of doubt. Because there are no mentors or visible representatives out there, that in itself becomes an obstacle for advancement. It's an example of systemic discrimination. Chika noted that many of her fellow students had been linking up with professionals in the field from an early age, yet because of the lack of visibility for people of colour, those inroads were just not available to her. She was constantly playing a game of catch-up just to reach the level of her classmates.

She expressed frustration about the tendency for academic structures to reroute black children away from university or pursuing a profession, at times channeling them into a stream below their capabilities. Her language is uncompromising when talking about the need to challenge this. She's a woman determined to do everything she can to dismantle oppressive forces in racist structures.

Instead of being intimidated and silenced by her encounters with racism, Chika has chosen to step up and become an advocate.

Building social capital can be done through mentorship, she insists. "It's incumbent on us to build that network of mentorship", says Chika, so students as young as 12 and 14 years old can have those insights into how the system works for them to achieve optimum success. It helps to make a dream tangible, to make it real. Black youth need to see people like us in those power circles and to create networks to provide them the pathways to getting where we are beyond that. She can't stress enough how vital it is to leverage opportunities when you've gotten a seat at the table. Being available, offering solidarity at many levels within an institution, it solidifies a sense of community and belonging.

She uses the phrase "minority tax" to describe how black professionals are inevitably called upon to do the diversity work for our institutions and organizations that they haven't done or don't want to do. It's frustrating. Yes, bring in someone with expertise to guide you to do the due diligence. But the tendency to just hire the person of colour to do the work isn't good enough. It's just a show unless there is a concerted effort to look within the organization and its leadership. What patterns are present that need to be unlearned?

And then Chika laid down this:

Being anti racist means acknowledging black people's contributions beyond diversity.

There is an overwhelming tendency to be seen as valued only in talk about diversity and inclusion. We are physicians. Call upon us for our expertise.

Chika rose to the limelight with the announcement that she would be class valedictorian. It resulted in dozens of media interviews within a very short time. Although her story served as a potent and positive outlet for the black community, it became yet another aspect of the BLM movement. What she found was this acute interest in her personal experiences with racism. She was asked to talk about her encounters in excruciating detail.

Chika was not down with having her black trauma turned into a sideshow, leaving her as a caricature. Her black suffering put on display made for good media, much like the George Floyd video and other examples of black people being lynched in broad daylight. And yet the pain of her trauma being turned into sensation was disregarded, she feels, because after experiencing the sheer callousness of how deep interviewers insisted on digging, once they got what they needed she was left having to work through being retraumatized.

Only once during the flurry of interviews was she actually compensated for her time and emotional expense, she admitted.

At that point I stepped in and told her that, yes, if she is going to be a leader, a voice, then she – we – have every authority to ask for what we want. If the media or organizations are going to call on black lived experiences, it's like any other form of expertise. People need to be financially compensated for that. Otherwise it's just taking advantage and getting something for nothing. There's a line in the sand with a lot of things and this is one of them.

Before we concluded our conversation, I told Chika I was straight up humbled by her dedication and I vowed to her that I would start up my own mentorship program, a glaring hole in my own commitment to leading unapologetically.

So I did.

Our program, based in Ottawa, now includes roughly 12 members ranging from high school aged to undergrad and grad students. We even have a couple of active medical students. We aim to meet at least once a month virtually or in person. Ultimately the aim is to guide them by providing tools to give them the best possible opportunities at all levels.

We help prepare students to get into med school, and for those who are already there, we give them the best opportunity to achieve their residency goals and offer insights to support them to the challenges of being black physicians.

The mentees are provided with opportunities to bolster their CVs, but we also offer talks from influential black clinicians. For those applying to med school, we even set up mock interviews.

I may be well into my own career, but it's never too late to learn from younger people with fresh minds and new ideas. Chika inspired me to do better.

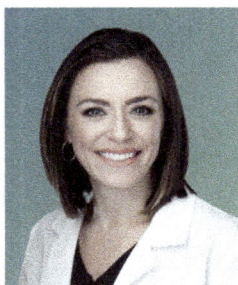

Unapologetically Engaged

Kali Dayton

When Kali Dayton joined my podcast for an episode on ICU patient outcomes, it was one of those great, great moments when I realized…yes!

Kali is a nurse practitioner and member of the Society of Critical Care Medicine in the United States. She and her team focus on early mobility and management of ICU delirium.

ICU delirium is a thing. It's caused when a patient has undergone long term sedation and they gain consciousness, only to have intense trauma from the experience. It's not that they are dreaming while sedated. They experience visions and scenarios that can be terrorizing and, to them, are very, very real. This can be accompanied by increased risks of PTSD and depression.

At the beginning of Kali's career, she was assigned to an ICU where she was asked to walk patients who were on ventilators. The practice in this particular unit was to allow intubated patients to wake up if there isn't any other complication requiring sedation. The patients would then be reoriented and allowed to communicate their needs, sometimes as early as a few hours after intubation.

Little did she know that this was an exception and not the norm.

When Kali was assigned to a different hospital, the ICU's environment was dramatically different. "Everyone looked like they were asleep," she told me. The patient she was assigned to was on a ventilator but sedated. When she asked the orientee nurse when she could get the patient up and for a walk, she was stared at in horror. "I quickly realized that that was the common perspective throughout the ICU, that I was the odd man out there."

So, she did it their way. She said she missed the human connection, witnessed patients being on ventilators for far longer, and saw outcomes more compromised.

The aha moment arrived when Kali sat beside an ICU survivor on a plane trip. When he learned she was an ICU nurse, he poured out a story about his sedation while on a ventilator. It shocked her.

"All he could fixate on was what it was like to be in the middle of a forest with his limbs nailed to the ground and trees were falling down on him and he couldn't run away. Demons were coming to the sky and a lot of things that he still couldn't talk about because he was so deeply traumatized. He was sobbing."

And that's when it struck her: to the patient those were not hallucinations. They were real. "He was psychologically scarred as if he physically lived through those scenarios." This man never returned to his career and had put his status down as "do not resuscitate" if he ever ended up back in the ICU because he didn't want to go through that horror ever again. He was in his 40s.

This conversation led Kali to interview ICU survivors and that's when she heard endless stories about the trauma of medically induced comas. It led to research about how harmful accepted practices are and what she found shocked her yet again: there was decades of research that had exposed the harm of long term sedation. Yet nothing had changed.

Our Resource Optimization team had put out a paper showing the financial impacts of ICU delirium. If we could reduce that, then money could then be diverted into more staffing, more resources, more physio, optimizing nutrition and other programs for increasing wellness. Kali mentioned that data shows that taking patients off sedation early reduces mortality by 68 percent.

Not only is it psychological torture, it's physically debilitating as well because of muscle breakdown. And because sedation isn't sleep, it leads to permanently reduced brain function. Whatever brought them into the ICU results in them leaving with chronic conditions.

Imagine being able to amplify getting well rather than staying debilitated.

I immediately told Kali we needed her to come and do regional rounds or a consultation, something that would have us more informed about how to make this happen.

We need this, because the pandemic's impact can't be ignored. So many of those people who have come off ventilators are going to need care for the rest of their lives. That chronic care echo is with us now and for years to come. If we can help people now and in the future to reduce that impact, to turn debilitation into rehabilitation, everyone wins.

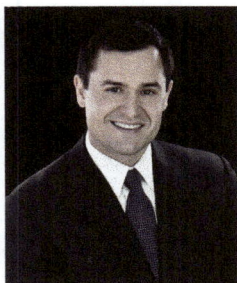

Unapologetically Fresh

Dr. Duane Hickling

It was only the fourth episode of "Solving Healthcare" I'd ever done, back before the COVID onslaught in 2020.

It was then I learned that the use of a medical scribe can improve a clinician's efficiency by 30 to 40 percent. That data is even more relevant now that we are in a post-pandemic healthcare crisis.

The information my colleague and friend Dr. Duane Hickling offered about the importance and efficiency of this service really resonates. And cost efficiency is, to me, not even the most vital part of it. It's the increased patient satisfaction and physician burnout that is avoided. You can't put a price on that.

Duane is a specialist in women's pelvic floor reconstruction. (As a side note, I was told that most of his patients wouldn't even need surgery if free physiotherapy had been available to them early on in their lives). Because his specialty is so focused, the amount of paperwork attached to each patient's chart is staggering. He told me that before he employed a medical scribe he was drowning in paperwork, frustrated over the level of care he was offering patients, and coming home exhausted and spent from having to take care of all the niggling details – finishing charts, ordering imaging, faxing prescriptions.

"I was gassed. I was tired," he said.

Part of the frustration in keeping medical records is that it's electronic, which means being glued to a screen even while having a patient consultation. But when a resident talked to him about using a scribe, it became a game changer.

Here's how it works. A physician can hire a scribe to record everything that is discussed and prescribed during a patient consultation. They are there in the room taking all the notes. Duane says he doesn't even have a pen in his hand now. Instead, he can sit and make eye contact with his patient, have a greater understanding of their needs, offer compassion, and have the peace of mind knowing that all the paperwork will be managed accurately.

That is just downright beautiful. Looking a patient in the eye? Something that basic changes everything. Doctors didn't come into this profession so they could spend their time staring at a screen. Duane said he was able to focus more on patient needs, listen to them, interact with them, and ultimately have a clear head for making the best possible decisions for them.

"My efficiency improved 30 to 40 percent," he said. That means seeing more patients and feeling good doing it.

We both have young families and when he told me he can go home at the end of his day feeling fresh, that just nailed it for me. Every little detail can grind away at a person, even things like ensuring nothing is misspelled in a report. For me it can lead to decision fatigue and well, burnout. So being able to go home, properly engage with my family and be 100 percent there for them?

There's no price tag for freshness. It's invaluable. Duane says it makes him feel like a better person overall while experiencing more job satisfaction.

But what about financial efficiency?

Duane said the investment return for him is about six to one. He pays for his scribe service out of his own practice, but because he can increase his billings, he's actually netting more.

Now think about how that would translate on a system-wide basis. Patient satisfaction improved, wait times reduced, and record accuracy maintained. It's win win.

I love this idea, especially since it plays right into the 80/20 principle I subscribe to – where 80 percent of results come from 20 percent of the effort. In a department like the ICU where I work, this would raise efficiency and cost savings exponentially. Again, it's not how much money you spend. It's how you spend it.

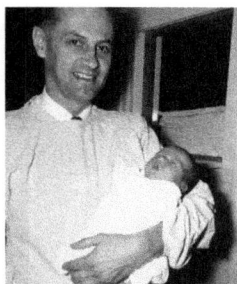

Unapologetically Principled

Dr. Gerhard Conradi

Growing up in Edmonton, Alberta, Canada, I suffered from childhood asthma, a tough condition for a hockey-playing kid who could never get enough time at the arena or in the minus 20 degrees of a prairie winter. I spent more time in the hospital than I care to remember.

What I do remember is how my pediatrician made me feel better. I'd be in a panic because I couldn't breathe, but then he would come in and put his soft hands on my chest, and I knew it would be okay. That presence, the calming nature he had, was healing. I'll never forget that.

I couldn't have possibly known that this doctor was a fifteenth generation physician. I couldn't have understood that this man's life was irrevocably changed because he dared to help someone he shouldn't have, someone from a group he was told to despise. To kill, even.

His name was Gerhard Conradi.

I didn't drift into medicine. I chose it at a young age. I wanted to do the same thing for other people, reach out with that calming presence that helps sick people heal. I wanted to be like Dr. Conradi.

What I didn't know was the price he had paid to stay true to who he was, or that I would someday have to face overwhelming pressure to act in a way that went against my own values. The price I have paid, albeit infinitely smaller than that of Dr. Conradi, has been in service to the vulnerable, regardless of who they were, what they looked like, how old they were or how much money they carried in their pockets.

Dr. Conradi's grandson, Nick, a physician himself, recounts the story of the momentous decision his Opi made in the war. With a few alterations, this is a post from Nick's blog, "Meditations of a Young Doctor."

Before immigrating to Canada, Gerhard Conradi studied medicine at the Friedrich Schiller University in Germany. Following his graduation in 1942, he was conscripted by the German military during the Second World War to serve as a wartime physician, leaving his wife, Karin, and three children to flee the country alone . . .

" . . . While on a patrol during the cold winter days of the war, my Opi came across an injured young soldier hiding in a snowbank, away from the passing German regiment. The man needed immediate medical attention and my Opi would be the only physician for miles. So, huddled in the snowbank alongside the stranger, my Opi decided to stay behind to help the man, an injured Russian soldier, the enemy.

The German soldiers had to go. My Opi had to stay. He spent hours tending to the young man, reassuring him that he would be alright – a guarantee made less with the confidence of its validity, and more for compassion's sake.

The two men would later be found by another passing regiment, this time from the Russian army. The Russians loaded the soldier onto a Russian vehicle. He was taken to the nearest military hospital. My Opi, however, would be less fortunate. He would spend two years imprisoned in a Russian prisoner of war camp, where he served as the camp's only physician – helped only by the camp's nurse.

The only way to get out was to create an illness that would induce the Russians to barter him for prisoners of their own. Desperate, he ingested charcoal from a friend's art kit and, predictably, fell ill. He would indeed be traded to the Germans during a prisoner exchange.

Reflecting on the event years later, my Opi would choose not to focus his attention on his imprisonment, but would instead wonder as to what came of the injured soldier he cared for. Instead of regretting his decision to care for the young man, which would ultimately lead to his imprisonment and prolonged absence from his family, he was reassured that his decision was one that led to the saving of a life."

Dr. Conradi made a decision to push past fear, to take another path that subverts the notion of us and them. He acted unapologetically. His vital decisions – to save another's life and to save his own – inspire me to do what's right, even if it means putting my own comfort aside.

Our choice is to stop favouring the haves over the have nots, the entitled over the disadvantaged, the powerful over the most vulnerable. Doing the right thing is never without consequence. You might be seen as holding unfashionable, unpopular opinions. You definitely will find yourself challenging your own biases, acknowledging that they exist, abandoning the moral high ground so many of us think we've already earned. You might not get promotions you feel you've earned. You might find yourself pilloried on social media but you will embolden countless others.

A man helped his enemy and for that was imprisoned. He poisoned himself to freedom. Years later a boy came to him, short of breath and left inspired, full of hope.

No single person, certainly not me, holds all the solutions but the solutions to our challenges have to involve every single person. A doctor named Gerhard Conradi taught me that and I know to my core that it's true.

Afterword - Unapologetically Happy

When I stepped up into a leadership role, it was because I was frustrated and angry about how things aren't right. I've given you several chapters about what's wrong and how I think we can fix it, but now that I'm concluding this journey with you I thought I'd share with you some really uplifting highlights of an interview I did in early 2023 with Neil Pasricha, who wrote The Book of Awesome.

I gotta tell you, it was one of the most enjoyable conversations I've had since starting the Kwadcast. Neil delivered a mountain of reasons why we need to seek gratitude, why we should work on our happiness before anything else, and what life should be all about.

This guy started out of the gate with a 15 minute long rant during which I swear he didn't actually breathe. I sat there chuckling and laughing, yet some of what this guy was talking about was really tragic – his wife had left him, he lost his house, his best friend took his own life. At that lowest point was when he started a blog listing 1,000 awesome things. When that picked up speed he began writing books, the first being the multi-million bestseller, The Book of Awesome. He went on (and on and on) about how finding awesomeness in everyday things matters, how it leads to a purposeful life, and how his life turned around and he's married, a dad, is happy driving a minivan and finally got to quit his job at Walmart because he's writing books about topics that matter to him.

As he was coming to the end of this masterful, epic 15 minutes of non-stop talking, he said he thinks of life as having won the lottery and that living in Canada is a bonus because we're always near the top of the rankings for quality of life – we trust our neighbours more, most of us have clean water, we can marry who we want to and other freedoms that are here for 40 million of us but not for most of those eight billion people who inhabit our world. And while social media and news media may want to punish us into thinking we aren't doing very well, it's just not true. And then he laid down this:

"We've got 30,000 days. That's it. Boom. We're done. So, how can we spend our lives as best we possibly can living the deepest, richest, most intentional lives possible?"

Neil, who can rattle off an encyclopedia of facts and stats in 30 seconds without skipping a beat, said our societal model has gotten it all wrong. The work hard, get successful and find happiness timeline is backwards. We need to be happy first and we must practice that daily. The rest comes later. Happy people live 10 years longer, he stated, so why not pursue that? And the key to finding what makes one happy is to just do The Thing.

"Action leads to motivation", said Neil.

Yes. That is straight up GOLD. You spent only five minutes at the gym? That's a win. You wrote something and it's awful? That's a win. Be in love with the process, not the goals. I felt a real kinship with Neil about this because it's one of my core beliefs.

As an ICU doctor and palliative care specialist, I can relate to this to my core. I see a lot of people in their final days and if there's one thing I am acutely aware of all the time it's that we're not here forever. We have to do stuff that's meaningful and maybe spend less time trying to please others. And say the stuff that needs to be said. I wish I could go back and have one last chat with my dad. However, I can take that lesson and apply it to my future.

What it all boils down to is this: I have three sons and an amazing wife who has my back and is a fabulous mother. My kids aren't poor, they have opportunity, they don't go hungry, and this is my shot at helping to raise good people who can be kind and compassionate and have tools for resilience. I want to teach them to live NOW because there are no guarantees, man.

And yes, I am happy. I'm as unapologetically being the best I can be with the 30,000 days I've been given.

I am, indeed, blessed.

www.ingramcontent.com/pod-product-compliance
Lightning Source LLC
Chambersburg PA
CBHW071212020426
42333CB00015B/1382